THIS JOURNAL BELONGS TO:

____

Active calories 2,000
40% carbs 800
30% Protein 600

PROGRESS TRACKER

30% fats 600

BMR 1314
Carb 1g = 4cal
Protein 1g = 4 cal
Fat = 1g = 9 cal

What to Track	Week 1	Week 2
Weight		
Chest		
Hips		
Arms		
Thighs		

What to Track	Week 3	Week 4	Week 5	Week 6
Weight				
Chest				
Hips				
Arms				
Thighs				

What to Track	Week 7	Week 8	Week 8	Week 10
Weight				
Chest				
Hips				
Arms				
Thighs				

What to Track	Week 11	Week 12	Week 13	Week 14
Weight				
Chest				
Hips				
Arms				
Thighs				

Date: 10-29-23

Fasting Day? Y N 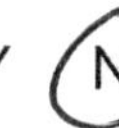

		Macros	
BREAKFAST	TJ PB bar	Protein	4 g
		Carbs	20 g
		Fat	8 g
		Calories	170
LUNCH	Egg sandwhich 1/2 milk cup bread - C 120, P 8, F 2, C 24 eggs - 144, 12, 10, 1 bacon - 240, 15, 21, 0	Protein	35 g
		Carbs	25 g
		Fat	33 g
		Calories	504
DINNER	Salmon Brussel Sprouts Couscous	Protein	
		Carbs	
		Fat	
		Calories	540
SNACKS	TJ Trail Mix TJ Cookies	Protein	5 g / 2 g
		Carbs	21 g / 25 g
		Fat	13 g / 6 g
		Calories	210 / 380

Hunger / Cravings

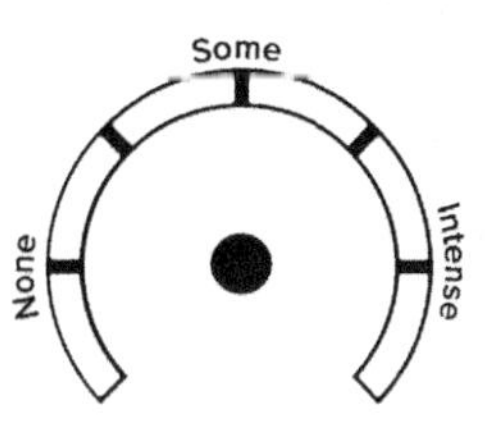

Hydration

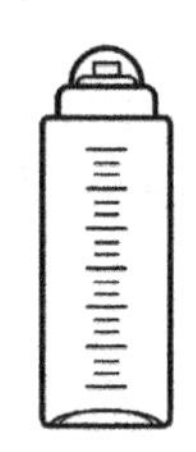

Today's Weight

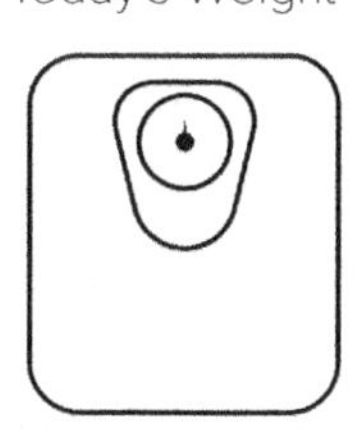

Notes / Observations

Bike - 30 miles

Gym - 40 mins

Today I Feel...

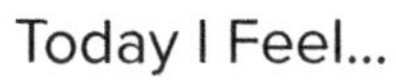

Sleep Quality

Sleep Time

Wake Time

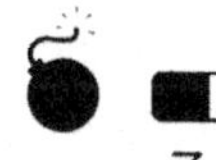 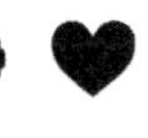

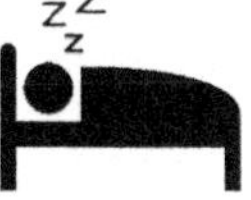

Date: 10-30-23 Fasting Day? Y (N)

		Macros	
BREAKFAST	Wheat slim and peanut butter	Protein	
		Carbs	
		Fat	
		Calories	
LUNCH	quinoi + brussel sprouts	Protein	
		Carbs	
		Fat	
		Calories	
DINNER	sushi	Protein	
		Carbs	
		Fat	
		Calories	600
SNACKS	Bag of trail mix some cashews handful of pretzels	Protein	
		Carbs	
		Fat	
		Calories	

Hunger / Cravings

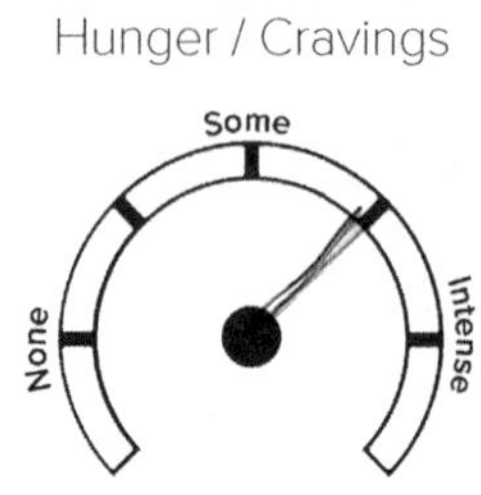

Hydration

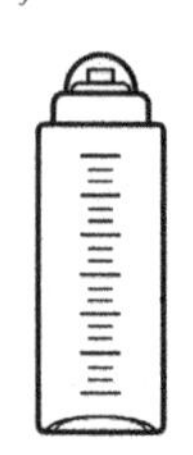

Today's Weight

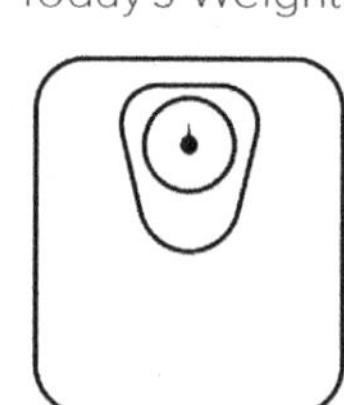

Notes / Observations

pushups - 50
sit ups - 50

Today I Feel...

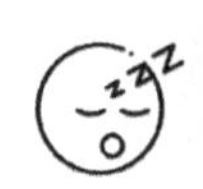

Sleep Quality

Sleep Time ____________

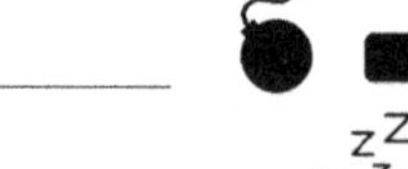

Wake Time ____________

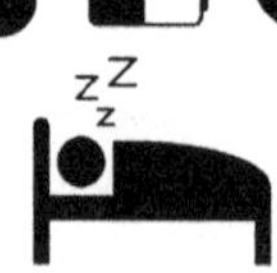

Date: ____________________ Fasting Day? Y N

		Macros	
BREAKFAST		Protein	
		Carbs	
		Fat	
		Calories	
		Macros	
LUNCH		Protein	
		Carbs	
		Fat	
		Calories	
		Macros	
DINNER		Protein	
		Carbs	
		Fat	
		Calories	
		Macros	
SNACKS		Protein	
		Carbs	
		Fat	
		Calories	

Hunger / Cravings

None Some Intense

Hydration

Today's Weight

Notes / Observations

Today I Feel...

Sleep Quality

Sleep Time

____

Wake Time

____

Date: ____________________ Fasting Day? Y N

		Macros	
BREAKFAST		Protein	
		Carbs	
		Fat	
		Calories	
LUNCH		Macros	
		Protein	
		Carbs	
		Fat	
		Calories	
DINNER		Macros	
		Protein	
		Carbs	
		Fat	
		Calories	
SNACKS		Macros	
		Protein	
		Carbs	
		Fat	
		Calories	

Hunger / Cravings

None Some Intense

Hydration

Today's Weight

Notes / Observations

Today I Feel...

Sleep Quality

Sleep Time ____________

Wake Time ____________

z z Z

Date: ______________________ Fasting Day? Y N

		Macros	
BREAKFAST		Protein	
		Carbs	
		Fat	
		Calories	
		Macros	
LUNCH		Protein	
		Carbs	
		Fat	
		Calories	
		Macros	
DINNER		Protein	
		Carbs	
		Fat	
		Calories	
		Macros	
SNACKS		Protein	
		Carbs	
		Fat	
		Calories	

Hunger / Cravings

None Some Intense

Hydration

Today's Weight

Notes / Observations

Today I Feel...

Sleep Quality

Sleep Time ____________

Wake Time ____________

Date: ______________________ Fasting Day? Y N

		Macros	
BREAKFAST		Protein	
		Carbs	
		Fat	
		Calories	
LUNCH		Macros	
		Protein	
		Carbs	
		Fat	
		Calories	
DINNER		Macros	
		Protein	
		Carbs	
		Fat	
		Calories	
SNACKS		Macros	
		Protein	
		Carbs	
		Fat	
		Calories	

Hunger / Cravings

None Some Intense

Hydration

Today's Weight

Notes / Observations

Today I Feel...

Sleep Quality

Sleep Time

Wake Time

Date: ____________________ Fasting Day? Y N

		Macros	
BREAKFAST		Protein	
		Carbs	
		Fat	
		Calories	
LUNCH		Macros	
		Protein	
		Carbs	
		Fat	
		Calories	
DINNER		Macros	
		Protein	
		Carbs	
		Fat	
		Calories	
SNACKS		Macros	
		Protein	
		Carbs	
		Fat	
		Calories	

Hunger / Cravings

None Some Intense

Hydration

Today's Weight

Notes / Observations

Today I Feel...

Sleep Quality

Sleep Time ____________

Wake Time ____________

Date: ______________________ Fasting Day? Y N

		Macros	
BREAKFAST		Protein	
		Carbs	
		Fat	
		Calories	
LUNCH		Macros	
		Protein	
		Carbs	
		Fat	
		Calories	
DINNER		Macros	
		Protein	
		Carbs	
		Fat	
		Calories	
SNACKS		Macros	
		Protein	
		Carbs	
		Fat	
		Calories	

Hunger / Cravings

None Some Intense

Hydration

Today's Weight

Notes / Observations

Today I Feel...

Sleep Quality

Sleep Time ______

Wake Time ______

Date: ______________________ Fasting Day? Y N

		Macros	
BREAKFAST		Protein	
		Carbs	
		Fat	
		Calories	
LUNCH		Macros	
		Protein	
		Carbs	
		Fat	
		Calories	
DINNER		Macros	
		Protein	
		Carbs	
		Fat	
		Calories	
SNACKS		Macros	
		Protein	
		Carbs	
		Fat	
		Calories	

Hunger / Cravings

None Some Intense

Hydration

Today's Weight

Notes / Observations

Today I Feel...

Sleep Quality

Sleep Time ____________

Wake Time ____________

Date: ______________________ Fasting Day? Y N

BREAKFAST		Macros	
		Protein	
		Carbs	
		Fat	
		Calories	
LUNCH		Macros	
		Protein	
		Carbs	
		Fat	
		Calories	
DINNER		Macros	
		Protein	
		Carbs	
		Fat	
		Calories	
SNACKS		Macros	
		Protein	
		Carbs	
		Fat	
		Calories	

Hunger / Cravings

None Some Intense

Hydration

Today's Weight

Notes / Observations

Today I Feel...

Sleep Quality

Sleep Time ____________

Wake Time ____________

Date: ____________________ Fasting Day? Y N

BREAKFAST		Macros	
		Protein	
		Carbs	
		Fat	
		Calories	
LUNCH		Macros	
		Protein	
		Carbs	
		Fat	
		Calories	
DINNER		Macros	
		Protein	
		Carbs	
		Fat	
		Calories	
SNACKS		Macros	
		Protein	
		Carbs	
		Fat	
		Calories	

Hunger / Cravings

None Some Intense

Hydration

Today's Weight

Notes / Observations

Today I Feel...

Sleep Quality

Sleep Time

Wake Time

Date: ______________________ Fasting Day? Y N

BREAKFAST		Macros	
		Protein	
		Carbs	
		Fat	
		Calories	
LUNCH		Macros	
		Protein	
		Carbs	
		Fat	
		Calories	
DINNER		Macros	
		Protein	
		Carbs	
		Fat	
		Calories	
SNACKS		Macros	
		Protein	
		Carbs	
		Fat	
		Calories	

Hunger / Cravings

None Some Intense

Hydration

Today's Weight

Notes / Observations

Today I Feel...

Sleep Quality

Sleep Time

____

Wake Time

____

Date: ____________________ Fasting Day? Y N

		Macros	
BREAKFAST		Protein	
		Carbs	
		Fat	
		Calories	
LUNCH		Macros	
		Protein	
		Carbs	
		Fat	
		Calories	
DINNER		Macros	
		Protein	
		Carbs	
		Fat	
		Calories	
SNACKS		Macros	
		Protein	
		Carbs	
		Fat	
		Calories	

Hunger / Cravings

None Some Intense

Hydration

Today's Weight

Notes / Observations

Today I Feel...

Sleep Quality

Sleep Time

Wake Time

Date: ______________________ Fasting Day? Y N

BREAKFAST		Macros	
		Protein	
		Carbs	
		Fat	
		Calories	
LUNCH		Macros	
		Protein	
		Carbs	
		Fat	
		Calories	
DINNER		Macros	
		Protein	
		Carbs	
		Fat	
		Calories	
SNACKS		Macros	
		Protein	
		Carbs	
		Fat	
		Calories	

Hunger / Cravings

None Some Intense

Hydration

Today's Weight

Notes / Observations

Today I Feel...

Sleep Quality

Sleep Time

____

Wake Time

____

Date: ______________________ Fasting Day? Y N

		Macros	
BREAKFAST		Protein	
		Carbs	
		Fat	
		Calories	
		Macros	
LUNCH		Protein	
		Carbs	
		Fat	
		Calories	
		Macros	
DINNER		Protein	
		Carbs	
		Fat	
		Calories	
		Macros	
SNACKS		Protein	
		Carbs	
		Fat	
		Calories	

Hunger / Cravings

None Some Intense

Hydration

Today's Weight

Notes / Observations

Today I Feel...

Sleep Quality

Sleep Time ____________

Wake Time ____________

Date: ______________________ Fasting Day? Y N

		Macros	
BREAKFAST		Protein	
		Carbs	
		Fat	
		Calories	
LUNCH		Macros	
		Protein	
		Carbs	
		Fat	
		Calories	
DINNER		Macros	
		Protein	
		Carbs	
		Fat	
		Calories	
SNACKS		Macros	
		Protein	
		Carbs	
		Fat	
		Calories	

Hunger / Cravings

None Some Intense

Hydration

Today's Weight

Notes / Observations

Today I Feel...

Sleep Quality

Sleep Time ______________

Wake Time ______________

Date: ______________________ Fasting Day? Y N

		Macros	
BREAKFAST		Protein	
		Carbs	
		Fat	
		Calories	
		Macros	
LUNCH		Protein	
		Carbs	
		Fat	
		Calories	
		Macros	
DINNER		Protein	
		Carbs	
		Fat	
		Calories	
		Macros	
SNACKS		Protein	
		Carbs	
		Fat	
		Calories	

Hunger / Cravings

None Some Intense

Hydration

Today's Weight

Notes / Observations

Today I Feel...

Sleep Quality

Sleep Time ____________

Wake Time ____________

Date: ____________________ Fasting Day? Y N

		Macros	
BREAKFAST		Protein	
		Carbs	
		Fat	
		Calories	
		Macros	
LUNCH		Protein	
		Carbs	
		Fat	
		Calories	
		Macros	
DINNER		Protein	
		Carbs	
		Fat	
		Calories	
		Macros	
SNACKS		Protein	
		Carbs	
		Fat	
		Calories	

Hunger / Cravings

None Some Intense

Hydration

Today's Weight

Notes / Observations

Today I Feel...

Sleep Quality

Sleep Time

Wake Time

Date: ______________________ Fasting Day? Y N

		Macros	
BREAKFAST		Protein	
		Carbs	
		Fat	
		Calories	
LUNCH		Macros	
		Protein	
		Carbs	
		Fat	
		Calories	
DINNER		Macros	
		Protein	
		Carbs	
		Fat	
		Calories	
SNACKS		Macros	
		Protein	
		Carbs	
		Fat	
		Calories	

Hunger / Cravings

None Some Intense

Hydration

Today's Weight

Notes / Observations

Today I Feel...

Sleep Quality

Sleep Time ____________

Wake Time ____________

Date: ______________________ Fasting Day? Y N

		Macros	
BREAKFAST		Protein	
		Carbs	
		Fat	
		Calories	
LUNCH		Macros	
		Protein	
		Carbs	
		Fat	
		Calories	
DINNER		Macros	
		Protein	
		Carbs	
		Fat	
		Calories	
SNACKS		Macros	
		Protein	
		Carbs	
		Fat	
		Calories	

Hunger / Cravings

None Some Intense

Hydration

Today's Weight

Notes / Observations

Today I Feel...

Sleep Quality

Sleep Time ____________

Wake Time ____________

Date: ______________________ Fasting Day? Y N

BREAKFAST		Macros	
		Protein	
		Carbs	
		Fat	
		Calories	
LUNCH		Macros	
		Protein	
		Carbs	
		Fat	
		Calories	
DINNER		Macros	
		Protein	
		Carbs	
		Fat	
		Calories	
SNACKS		Macros	
		Protein	
		Carbs	
		Fat	
		Calories	

Hunger / Cravings

None Some Intense

Hydration

Today's Weight

Notes / Observations

....

....

....

....

....

....

....

....

....

....

Today I Feel...

Sleep Quality

Sleep Time

____

Wake Time

____

Date: ______________________ Fasting Day? Y N

BREAKFAST		Macros	
		Protein	
		Carbs	
		Fat	
		Calories	
LUNCH		Macros	
		Protein	
		Carbs	
		Fat	
		Calories	
DINNER		Macros	
		Protein	
		Carbs	
		Fat	
		Calories	
SNACKS		Macros	
		Protein	
		Carbs	
		Fat	
		Calories	

Hunger / Cravings

None Some Intense

Hydration

Today's Weight

Notes / Observations

Today I Feel...

Sleep Quality

Sleep Time

____

Wake Time

____

Date: ______________________ Fasting Day? Y N

		Macros	
BREAKFAST		Protein	
		Carbs	
		Fat	
		Calories	
LUNCH		Macros	
		Protein	
		Carbs	
		Fat	
		Calories	
DINNER		Macros	
		Protein	
		Carbs	
		Fat	
		Calories	
SNACKS		Macros	
		Protein	
		Carbs	
		Fat	
		Calories	

Hunger / Cravings

None Some Intense

Hydration

Today's Weight

Notes / Observations

Today I Feel...

Sleep Quality

Sleep Time

____

Wake Time

____

Date: ______________________ Fasting Day? Y N

		Macros	
BREAKFAST		Protein	
		Carbs	
		Fat	
		Calories	
LUNCH		Macros	
		Protein	
		Carbs	
		Fat	
		Calories	
DINNER		Macros	
		Protein	
		Carbs	
		Fat	
		Calories	
SNACKS		Macros	
		Protein	
		Carbs	
		Fat	
		Calories	

Hunger / Cravings

None Some Intense

Hydration

Today's Weight

Notes / Observations

Today I Feel...

Sleep Quality

Sleep Time ______________

Wake Time ______________

Date: ______________________ Fasting Day? Y N

		Macros	
BREAKFAST		Protein	
		Carbs	
		Fat	
		Calories	
LUNCH		Macros	
		Protein	
		Carbs	
		Fat	
		Calories	
DINNER		Macros	
		Protein	
		Carbs	
		Fat	
		Calories	
SNACKS		Macros	
		Protein	
		Carbs	
		Fat	
		Calories	

Hunger / Cravings

None Some Intense

Hydration

Today's Weight

Notes / Observations

Today I Feel...

Sleep Quality

Sleep Time

Wake Time

Date: ____________________ Fasting Day? Y N

BREAKFAST		Macros	
		Protein	
		Carbs	
		Fat	
		Calories	
LUNCH		Macros	
		Protein	
		Carbs	
		Fat	
		Calories	
DINNER		Macros	
		Protein	
		Carbs	
		Fat	
		Calories	
SNACKS		Macros	
		Protein	
		Carbs	
		Fat	
		Calories	

Hunger / Cravings

None Some Intense

Hydration

Today's Weight

Notes / Observations

Today I Feel...

Sleep Quality

Sleep Time

Wake Time

Date: ____________________ Fasting Day? Y N

		Macros	
BREAKFAST		Protein	
		Carbs	
		Fat	
		Calories	
LUNCH		Macros	
		Protein	
		Carbs	
		Fat	
		Calories	
DINNER		Macros	
		Protein	
		Carbs	
		Fat	
		Calories	
SNACKS		Macros	
		Protein	
		Carbs	
		Fat	
		Calories	

Hunger / Cravings

None Some Intense

Hydration

Today's Weight

Notes / Observations

Today I Feel...

Sleep Quality

Sleep Time

Wake Time

Date: ____________________ Fasting Day? Y N

		Macros	
BREAKFAST		Protein	
		Carbs	
		Fat	
		Calories	
LUNCH		Macros	
		Protein	
		Carbs	
		Fat	
		Calories	
DINNER		Macros	
		Protein	
		Carbs	
		Fat	
		Calories	
SNACKS		Macros	
		Protein	
		Carbs	
		Fat	
		Calories	

Hunger / Cravings

None Some Intense

Hydration

Today's Weight

Notes / Observations

Today I Feel...

Sleep Quality

Sleep Time

Wake Time

Date: ____________________ Fasting Day? Y N

		Macros	
BREAKFAST		Protein	
		Carbs	
		Fat	
		Calories	
		Macros	
LUNCH		Protein	
		Carbs	
		Fat	
		Calories	
		Macros	
DINNER		Protein	
		Carbs	
		Fat	
		Calories	
		Macros	
SNACKS		Protein	
		Carbs	
		Fat	
		Calories	

Hunger / Cravings

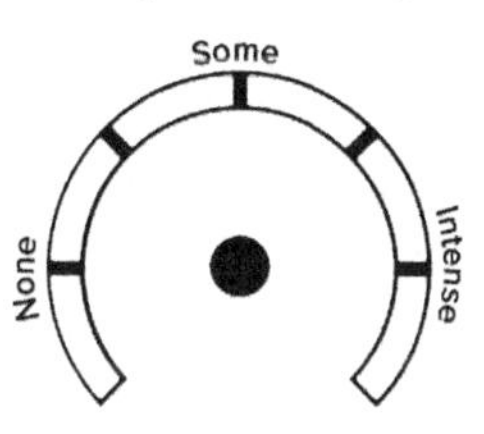

Hydration

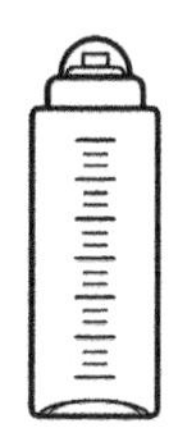

Today's Weight

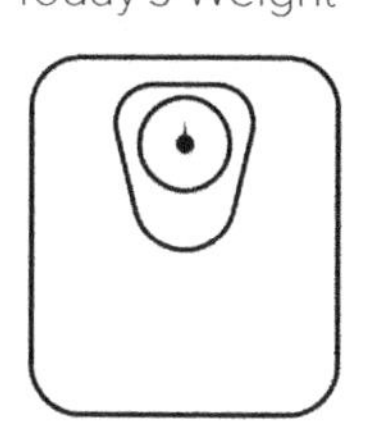

Notes / Observations

Today I Feel...

Sleep Quality

Sleep Time ____________

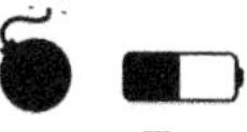

Wake Time ____________

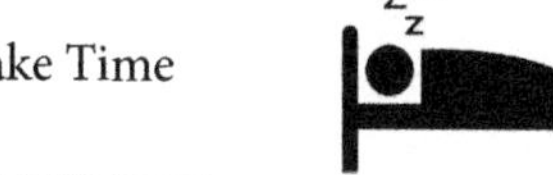

Date: ____________________ Fasting Day? Y N

		Macros	
BREAKFAST		Protein	
		Carbs	
		Fat	
		Calories	
LUNCH		Macros	
		Protein	
		Carbs	
		Fat	
		Calories	
DINNER		Macros	
		Protein	
		Carbs	
		Fat	
		Calories	
SNACKS		Macros	
		Protein	
		Carbs	
		Fat	
		Calories	

Hunger / Cravings

None Some Intense

Hydration

Today's Weight

Notes / Observations

Today I Feel...

Sleep Quality

Sleep Time

Wake Time

Date: ____________________ Fasting Day? Y N

		Macros	
BREAKFAST		Protein	
		Carbs	
		Fat	
		Calories	
LUNCH		Macros	
		Protein	
		Carbs	
		Fat	
		Calories	
DINNER		Macros	
		Protein	
		Carbs	
		Fat	
		Calories	
SNACKS		Macros	
		Protein	
		Carbs	
		Fat	
		Calories	

Hunger / Cravings

None Some Intense

Hydration

Today's Weight

Notes / Observations

Today I Feel...

Sleep Quality

Sleep Time

Wake Time

Date: ______________________ Fasting Day? Y N

BREAKFAST		Macros	
		Protein	
		Carbs	
		Fat	
		Calories	
LUNCH		Macros	
		Protein	
		Carbs	
		Fat	
		Calories	
DINNER		Macros	
		Protein	
		Carbs	
		Fat	
		Calories	
SNACKS		Macros	
		Protein	
		Carbs	
		Fat	
		Calories	

Hunger / Cravings

None Some Intense

Hydration

Today's Weight

Notes / Observations

Today I Feel...

Sleep Quality

Sleep Time ____________

Wake Time ____________

Date: ______________________ Fasting Day? Y N

		Macros	
BREAKFAST		Protein	
		Carbs	
		Fat	
		Calories	
LUNCH		Macros	
		Protein	
		Carbs	
		Fat	
		Calories	
DINNER		Macros	
		Protein	
		Carbs	
		Fat	
		Calories	
SNACKS		Macros	
		Protein	
		Carbs	
		Fat	
		Calories	

Hunger / Cravings

None Some Intense

Hydration

Today's Weight

Notes / Observations

Today I Feel...

Sleep Quality

Sleep Time

Wake Time

Date: ______________________ Fasting Day? Y N

BREAKFAST		Macros	
		Protein	
		Carbs	
		Fat	
		Calories	
LUNCH		Macros	
		Protein	
		Carbs	
		Fat	
		Calories	
DINNER		Macros	
		Protein	
		Carbs	
		Fat	
		Calories	
SNACKS		Macros	
		Protein	
		Carbs	
		Fat	
		Calories	

Hunger / Cravings

None Some Intense

Hydration

Today's Weight

Notes / Observations

Today I Feel...

Sleep Quality

Sleep Time ______

Wake Time ______

Date: ______________________ Fasting Day? Y N

		Macros	
BREAKFAST		Protein	
		Carbs	
		Fat	
		Calories	
LUNCH		Macros	
		Protein	
		Carbs	
		Fat	
		Calories	
DINNER		Macros	
		Protein	
		Carbs	
		Fat	
		Calories	
SNACKS		Macros	
		Protein	
		Carbs	
		Fat	
		Calories	

Hunger / Cravings

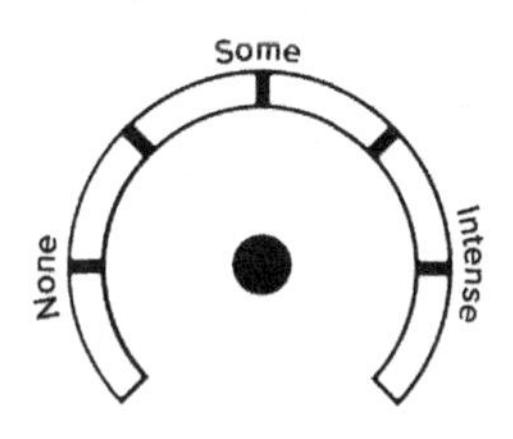

Hydration

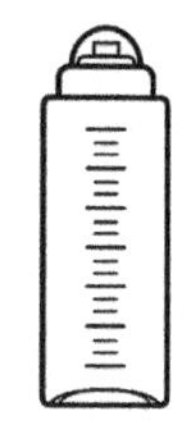

Today's Weight

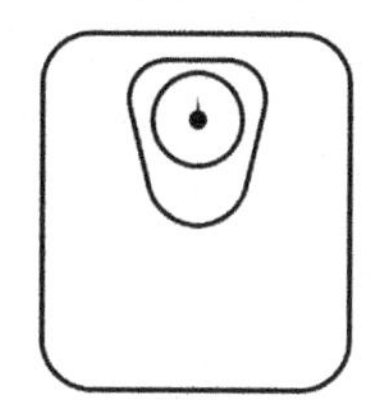

Notes / Observations

....

....

....

....

....

....

....

....

....

....

Today I Feel...

Sleep Quality

Sleep Time

____

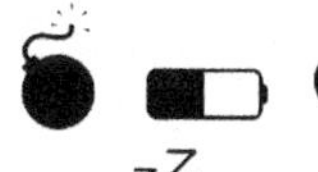

Wake Time

____

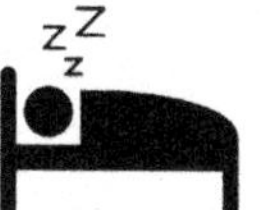

Date: ______________________ Fasting Day? Y N

		Macros	
BREAKFAST		Protein	
		Carbs	
		Fat	
		Calories	
LUNCH		Macros	
		Protein	
		Carbs	
		Fat	
		Calories	
DINNER		Macros	
		Protein	
		Carbs	
		Fat	
		Calories	
SNACKS		Macros	
		Protein	
		Carbs	
		Fat	
		Calories	

Hunger / Cravings

None Some Intense

Hydration

Today's Weight

Notes / Observations

Today I Feel...

Sleep Quality

Sleep Time

Wake Time

Date: ______________________ Fasting Day? Y N

BREAKFAST		Macros	
		Protein	
		Carbs	
		Fat	
		Calories	
LUNCH		Macros	
		Protein	
		Carbs	
		Fat	
		Calories	
DINNER		Macros	
		Protein	
		Carbs	
		Fat	
		Calories	
SNACKS		Macros	
		Protein	
		Carbs	
		Fat	
		Calories	

Hunger / Cravings

None Some Intense

Hydration

Today's Weight

Notes / Observations

Today I Feel...

Sleep Quality

Sleep Time

____

Wake Time

____

Date: ______________________ Fasting Day? Y N

		Macros	
BREAKFAST		Protein	
		Carbs	
		Fat	
		Calories	
LUNCH		Macros	
		Protein	
		Carbs	
		Fat	
		Calories	
DINNER		Macros	
		Protein	
		Carbs	
		Fat	
		Calories	
SNACKS		Macros	
		Protein	
		Carbs	
		Fat	
		Calories	

Hunger / Cravings

None Some Intense

Hydration

Today's Weight

Notes / Observations

Today I Feel...

Sleep Quality

Sleep Time ______

Wake Time ______

Date: ____________________ Fasting Day? Y N

BREAKFAST		Macros	
		Protein	
		Carbs	
		Fat	
		Calories	
LUNCH		Macros	
		Protein	
		Carbs	
		Fat	
		Calories	
DINNER		Macros	
		Protein	
		Carbs	
		Fat	
		Calories	
SNACKS		Macros	
		Protein	
		Carbs	
		Fat	
		Calories	

Hunger / Cravings

None Some Intense

Hydration

Today's Weight

Notes / Observations

Today I Feel...

Sleep Quality

Sleep Time

Wake Time

Date: ______________________ Fasting Day? Y N

		Macros	
BREAKFAST		Protein	
		Carbs	
		Fat	
		Calories	
		Macros	
LUNCH		Protein	
		Carbs	
		Fat	
		Calories	
		Macros	
DINNER		Protein	
		Carbs	
		Fat	
		Calories	
		Macros	
SNACKS		Protein	
		Carbs	
		Fat	
		Calories	

Hunger / Cravings

None Some Intense

Hydration

Today's Weight

Notes / Observations

Today I Feel...

Sleep Quality

Sleep Time ______________

Wake Time ______________

Date: ______________________ Fasting Day? Y N

		Macros	
BREAKFAST		Protein	
		Carbs	
		Fat	
		Calories	
LUNCH		Macros	
		Protein	
		Carbs	
		Fat	
		Calories	
DINNER		Macros	
		Protein	
		Carbs	
		Fat	
		Calories	
SNACKS		Macros	
		Protein	
		Carbs	
		Fat	
		Calories	

Hunger / Cravings

None Some Intense

Hydration

Today's Weight

Notes / Observations

....

....

....

....

....

....

....

....

....

....

Today I Feel...

Sleep Quality

Sleep Time

____

Wake Time

____

Date: ____________________ Fasting Day? Y N

		Macros	
BREAKFAST		Protein	
		Carbs	
		Fat	
		Calories	
LUNCH		Macros	
		Protein	
		Carbs	
		Fat	
		Calories	
DINNER		Macros	
		Protein	
		Carbs	
		Fat	
		Calories	
SNACKS		Macros	
		Protein	
		Carbs	
		Fat	
		Calories	

Hunger / Cravings

None Some Intense

Hydration

Today's Weight

Notes / Observations

Today I Feel...

Sleep Quality

Sleep Time

Wake Time

Date: ____________________ Fasting Day? Y N

		Macros	
BREAKFAST		Protein	
		Carbs	
		Fat	
		Calories	
LUNCH		Macros	
		Protein	
		Carbs	
		Fat	
		Calories	
DINNER		Macros	
		Protein	
		Carbs	
		Fat	
		Calories	
SNACKS		Macros	
		Protein	
		Carbs	
		Fat	
		Calories	

Hunger / Cravings

None Some Intense

Hydration

Today's Weight

Notes / Observations

....

....

....

....

....

....

....

....

....

....

Today I Feel...

Sleep Quality

Sleep Time ____________

Wake Time ____________

Date: ____________________ Fasting Day? Y N

		Macros	
BREAKFAST		Protein	
		Carbs	
		Fat	
		Calories	
LUNCH		Macros	
		Protein	
		Carbs	
		Fat	
		Calories	
DINNER		Macros	
		Protein	
		Carbs	
		Fat	
		Calories	
SNACKS		Macros	
		Protein	
		Carbs	
		Fat	
		Calories	

Hunger / Cravings

None Some Intense

Hydration

Today's Weight

Notes / Observations

Today I Feel...

Sleep Quality

Sleep Time

Wake Time

Date: ______________________ Fasting Day? Y N

		Macros	
BREAKFAST		Protein	
		Carbs	
		Fat	
		Calories	
LUNCH		Macros	
		Protein	
		Carbs	
		Fat	
		Calories	
DINNER		Macros	
		Protein	
		Carbs	
		Fat	
		Calories	
SNACKS		Macros	
		Protein	
		Carbs	
		Fat	
		Calories	

Hunger / Cravings

None Some Intense

Hydration

Today's Weight

Notes / Observations

Today I Feel...

Sleep Quality

Sleep Time

____

Wake Time

____

Date: ____________________ Fasting Day? Y N

BREAKFAST		Macros	
		Protein	
		Carbs	
		Fat	
		Calories	
LUNCH		Macros	
		Protein	
		Carbs	
		Fat	
		Calories	
DINNER		Macros	
		Protein	
		Carbs	
		Fat	
		Calories	
SNACKS		Macros	
		Protein	
		Carbs	
		Fat	
		Calories	

Hunger / Cravings

None Some Intense

Hydration

Today's Weight

Notes / Observations

Today I Feel...

Sleep Quality

Sleep Time

Wake Time

Date: ______________________ Fasting Day? Y N

		Macros	
BREAKFAST		Protein	
		Carbs	
		Fat	
		Calories	
LUNCH		Macros	
		Protein	
		Carbs	
		Fat	
		Calories	
DINNER		Macros	
		Protein	
		Carbs	
		Fat	
		Calories	
SNACKS		Macros	
		Protein	
		Carbs	
		Fat	
		Calories	

Hunger / Cravings

None Some Intense

Hydration

Today's Weight

Notes / Observations

Today I Feel...

Sleep Quality

Sleep Time ____________

Wake Time ____________

Date: ______________________ Fasting Day? Y N

		Macros	
BREAKFAST		Protein	
		Carbs	
		Fat	
		Calories	
LUNCH		Macros	
		Protein	
		Carbs	
		Fat	
		Calories	
DINNER		Macros	
		Protein	
		Carbs	
		Fat	
		Calories	
SNACKS		Macros	
		Protein	
		Carbs	
		Fat	
		Calories	

Hunger / Cravings

None Some Intense

Hydration

Today's Weight

Notes / Observations

Today I Feel...

Sleep Quality

Sleep Time

Wake Time

Date: ______________________ Fasting Day? Y N

		Macros	
BREAKFAST		Protein	
		Carbs	
		Fat	
		Calories	
LUNCH		Macros	
		Protein	
		Carbs	
		Fat	
		Calories	
DINNER		Macros	
		Protein	
		Carbs	
		Fat	
		Calories	
SNACKS		Macros	
		Protein	
		Carbs	
		Fat	
		Calories	

Hunger / Cravings

None Some Intense

Hydration

Today's Weight

Notes / Observations

Today I Feel...

Sleep Quality

Sleep Time

Wake Time

Date: ______________________ Fasting Day? Y N

		Macros	
BREAKFAST		Protein	
		Carbs	
		Fat	
		Calories	
LUNCH		Macros	
		Protein	
		Carbs	
		Fat	
		Calories	
DINNER		Macros	
		Protein	
		Carbs	
		Fat	
		Calories	
SNACKS		Macros	
		Protein	
		Carbs	
		Fat	
		Calories	

Hunger / Cravings

None Some Intense

Hydration

Today's Weight

Notes / Observations

Today I Feel...

Sleep Quality

Sleep Time ____________

Wake Time ____________

Date: ______________________ Fasting Day? Y N

		Macros	
BREAKFAST		Protein	
		Carbs	
		Fat	
		Calories	
LUNCH		Macros	
		Protein	
		Carbs	
		Fat	
		Calories	
DINNER		Macros	
		Protein	
		Carbs	
		Fat	
		Calories	
SNACKS		Macros	
		Protein	
		Carbs	
		Fat	
		Calories	

Hunger / Cravings

None Some Intense

Hydration

Today's Weight

Notes / Observations

Today I Feel...

Sleep Quality

Sleep Time ______

Wake Time ______

Date: ____________________ Fasting Day? Y N

		Macros	
BREAKFAST		Protein	
		Carbs	
		Fat	
		Calories	
LUNCH		Macros	
		Protein	
		Carbs	
		Fat	
		Calories	
DINNER		Macros	
		Protein	
		Carbs	
		Fat	
		Calories	
SNACKS		Macros	
		Protein	
		Carbs	
		Fat	
		Calories	

Hunger / Cravings

Some

None

Intense

Hydration

Today's Weight

Notes / Observations

Today I Feel...

Sleep Quality

Sleep Time

Wake Time

Date: ______________________ Fasting Day? Y N

		Macros	
BREAKFAST		Protein	
		Carbs	
		Fat	
		Calories	
		Macros	
LUNCH		Protein	
		Carbs	
		Fat	
		Calories	
		Macros	
DINNER		Protein	
		Carbs	
		Fat	
		Calories	
		Macros	
SNACKS		Protein	
		Carbs	
		Fat	
		Calories	

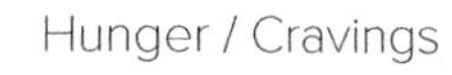

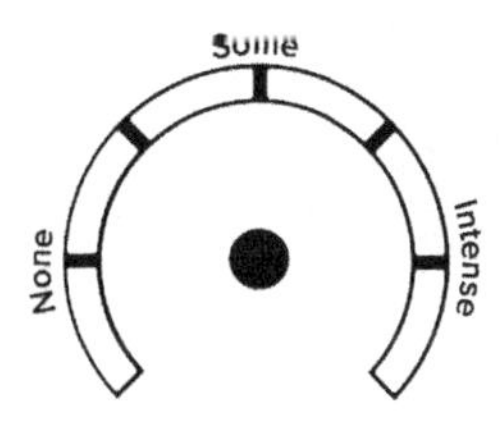

Hydration

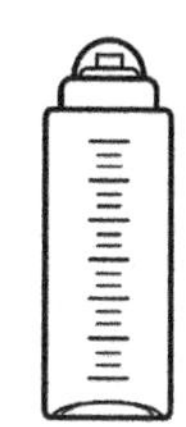

Today's Weight

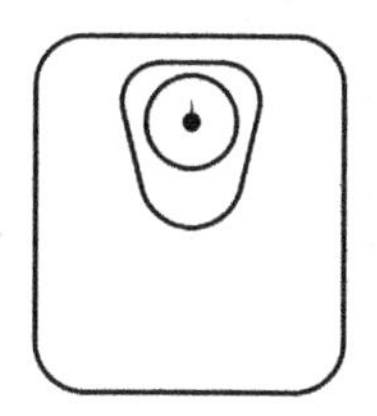

Notes / Observations

....

....

....

....

....

....

....

....

....

....

Today I Feel...

Sleep Quality

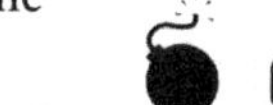

____

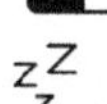

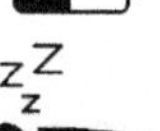

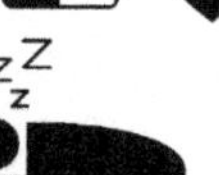

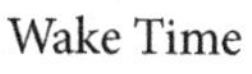

____

Date: ______________________ Fasting Day? Y N

BREAKFAST		MACROS	
		Protein	
		Carbs	
		Fat	
		Calories	
LUNCH		MACROS	
		Protein	
		Carbs	
		Fat	
		Calories	
DINNER		MACROS	
		Protein	
		Carbs	
		Fat	
		Calories	
SNACKS		MACROS	
		Protein	
		Carbs	
		Fat	
		Calories	

Hunger / Cravings

None Some Intense

Hydration

Today's Weight

Notes / Observations

Today I Feel...

Sleep Quality

Sleep Time

____

Wake Time

____

Date: ______________________ Fasting Day? Y N

		Macros	
BREAKFAST		Protein	
		Carbs	
		Fat	
		Calories	
		Macros	
LUNCH		Protein	
		Carbs	
		Fat	
		Calories	
		Macros	
DINNER		Protein	
		Carbs	
		Fat	
		Calories	
		Macros	
SNACKS		Protein	
		Carbs	
		Fat	
		Calories	

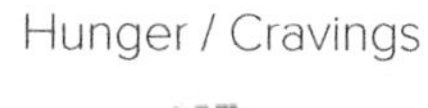

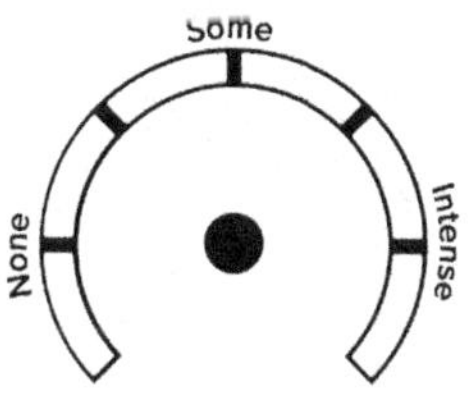

Hydration

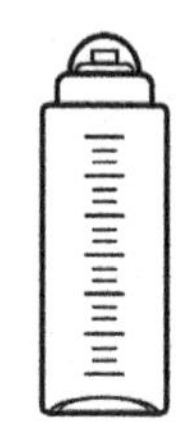

Today's Weight

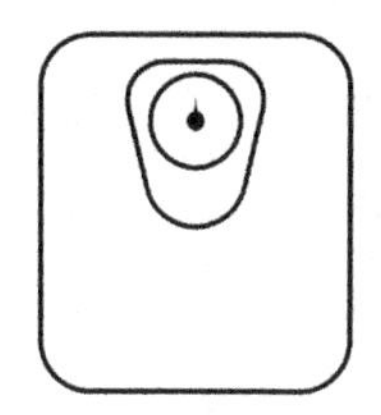

Notes / Observations

....

....

....

....

....

....

....

....

....

....

Today I Feel...

Sleep Quality

Sleep Time

____

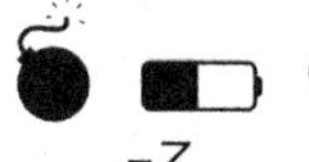

Wake Time

____

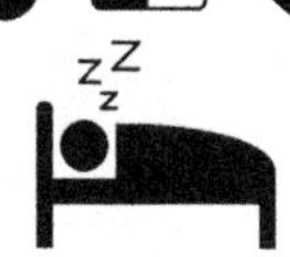

Date: ______________________ Fasting Day? Y N

		Macros	
BREAKFAST		Protein	
		Carbs	
		Fat	
		Calories	
LUNCH		Macros	
		Protein	
		Carbs	
		Fat	
		Calories	
DINNER		Macros	
		Protein	
		Carbs	
		Fat	
		Calories	
SNACKS		Macros	
		Protein	
		Carbs	
		Fat	
		Calories	

Hunger / Cravings

None Some Intense

Hydration

Today's Weight

Notes / Observations

Today I Feel...

Sleep Quality

Sleep Time ____________

Wake Time ____________

Date: ______________________ Fasting Day? Y N

		Macros	
BREAKFAST		Protein	
		Carbs	
		Fat	
		Calories	
LUNCH		Macros	
		Protein	
		Carbs	
		Fat	
		Calories	
DINNER		Macros	
		Protein	
		Carbs	
		Fat	
		Calories	
SNACKS		Macros	
		Protein	
		Carbs	
		Fat	
		Calories	

Hunger / Cravings

None Some Intense

Hydration

Today's Weight

Notes / Observations

Today I Feel...

Sleep Quality

Sleep Time ______

Wake Time ______

Date: ______________________ Fasting Day? Y N

BREAKFAST		Macros	
		Protein	
		Carbs	
		Fat	
		Calories	
LUNCH		Macros	
		Protein	
		Carbs	
		Fat	
		Calories	
DINNER		Macros	
		Protein	
		Carbs	
		Fat	
		Calories	
SNACKS		Macros	
		Protein	
		Carbs	
		Fat	
		Calories	

Hunger / Cravings

None Some Intense

Hydration

Today's Weight

Notes / Observations

Today I Feel...

Sleep Quality

Sleep Time ____________

Wake Time ____________

Date: ______________________ Fasting Day? Y N

		Macros	
BREAKFAST		Protein	
		Carbs	
		Fat	
		Calories	
LUNCH		Macros	
		Protein	
		Carbs	
		Fat	
		Calories	
DINNER		Macros	
		Protein	
		Carbs	
		Fat	
		Calories	
SNACKS		Macros	
		Protein	
		Carbs	
		Fat	
		Calories	

Hunger / Cravings

None Some Intense

Hydration

Today's Weight

Notes / Observations

Today I Feel...

Sleep Quality

Sleep Time ____________

Wake Time ____________

Date: ______________________ Fasting Day? Y N

		Macros	
BREAKFAST		Protein	
		Carbs	
		Fat	
		Calories	
		Macros	
LUNCH		Protein	
		Carbs	
		Fat	
		Calories	
		Macros	
DINNER		Protein	
		Carbs	
		Fat	
		Calories	
		Macros	
SNACKS		Protein	
		Carbs	
		Fat	
		Calories	

Hunger / Cravings

None Some Intense

Hydration

Today's Weight

Notes / Observations

Today I Feel...

Sleep Quality

Sleep Time ______

Wake Time ______

Date: ______________________ Fasting Day? Y N

		Macros	
BREAKFAST		Protein	
		Carbs	
		Fat	
		Calories	
LUNCH		Macros	
		Protein	
		Carbs	
		Fat	
		Calories	
DINNER		Macros	
		Protein	
		Carbs	
		Fat	
		Calories	
SNACKS		Macros	
		Protein	
		Carbs	
		Fat	
		Calories	

Hunger / Cravings

None Some Intense

Hydration

Today's Weight

Notes / Observations

Today I Feel...

Sleep Quality

Sleep Time

Wake Time

Date: ______________________ Fasting Day? Y N

		Macros	
BREAKFAST		Protein	
		Carbs	
		Fat	
		Calories	
LUNCH		Macros	
		Protein	
		Carbs	
		Fat	
		Calories	
DINNER		Macros	
		Protein	
		Carbs	
		Fat	
		Calories	
SNACKS		Macros	
		Protein	
		Carbs	
		Fat	
		Calories	

Hunger / Cravings

None Some Intense

Hydration

Today's Weight

Notes / Observations

Today I Feel...

Sleep Quality

Sleep Time

____

Wake Time

____

Date: ______________________ Fasting Day? Y N

BREAKFAST		Macros	
		Protein	
		Carbs	
		Fat	
		Calories	
LUNCH		Macros	
		Protein	
		Carbs	
		Fat	
		Calories	
DINNER		Macros	
		Protein	
		Carbs	
		Fat	
		Calories	
SNACKS		Macros	
		Protein	
		Carbs	
		Fat	
		Calories	

Hunger / Cravings

None Some Intense

Hydration

Today's Weight

Notes / Observations

Today I Feel...

Sleep Quality

Sleep Time

Wake Time

Date: ______________________ Fasting Day? Y N

		Macros	
BREAKFAST		Protein	
		Carbs	
		Fat	
		Calories	
LUNCH		Macros	
		Protein	
		Carbs	
		Fat	
		Calories	
DINNER		Macros	
		Protein	
		Carbs	
		Fat	
		Calories	
SNACKS		Macros	
		Protein	
		Carbs	
		Fat	
		Calories	

Hunger / Cravings

None Some Intense

Hydration

Today's Weight

Notes / Observations

Today I Feel...

Sleep Quality

Sleep Time

Wake Time

Date: ______________________ Fasting Day? Y N

		Macros	
BREAKFAST		Protein	
		Carbs	
		Fat	
		Calories	
LUNCH		Macros	
		Protein	
		Carbs	
		Fat	
		Calories	
DINNER		Macros	
		Protein	
		Carbs	
		Fat	
		Calories	
SNACKS		Macros	
		Protein	
		Carbs	
		Fat	
		Calories	

Hunger / Cravings

None Some Intense

Hydration

Today's Weight

Notes / Observations

Today I Feel...

Sleep Quality

Sleep Time

Wake Time

Date: ______________________ Fasting Day? Y N

		Macros	
BREAKFAST		Protein	
		Carbs	
		Fat	
		Calories	
		Macros	
LUNCH		Protein	
		Carbs	
		Fat	
		Calories	
		Macros	
DINNER		Protein	
		Carbs	
		Fat	
		Calories	
		Macros	
SNACKS		Protein	
		Carbs	
		Fat	
		Calories	

Hunger / Cravings

None Some Intense

Hydration

Today's Weight

Notes / Observations

Today I Feel...

Sleep Quality

Sleep Time

Wake Time

Date: ______________________ Fasting Day? Y N

		Macros	
BREAKFAST		Protein	
		Carbs	
		Fat	
		Calories	
LUNCH		Macros	
		Protein	
		Carbs	
		Fat	
		Calories	
DINNER		Macros	
		Protein	
		Carbs	
		Fat	
		Calories	
SNACKS		Macros	
		Protein	
		Carbs	
		Fat	
		Calories	

Hunger / Cravings

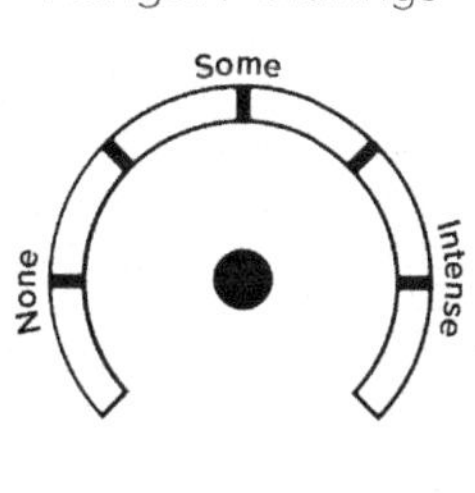

Hydration

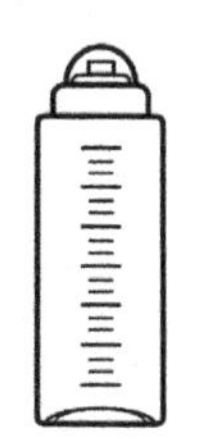

Today's Weight

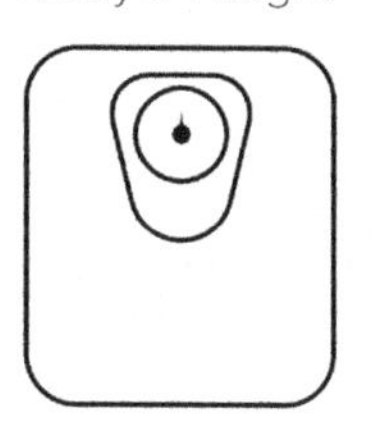

Notes / Observations

....

....

....

....

....

....

....

....

....

....

Today I Feel...

Sleep Quality

Sleep Time

____

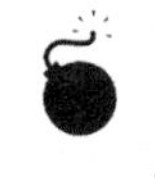

Wake Time

____

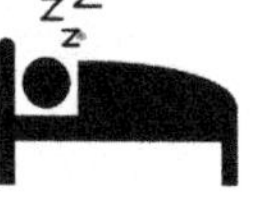

Date: ______________________ Fasting Day? Y N

		Macros	
BREAKFAST		Protein	
		Carbs	
		Fat	
		Calories	
LUNCH		Macros	
		Protein	
		Carbs	
		Fat	
		Calories	
DINNER		Macros	
		Protein	
		Carbs	
		Fat	
		Calories	
SNACKS		Macros	
		Protein	
		Carbs	
		Fat	
		Calories	

Hunger / Cravings

None Some Intense

Hydration

Today's Weight

Notes / Observations

....

....

....

....

....

....

....

....

....

....

Today I Feel...

Sleep Quality

Sleep Time

____

Wake Time

____

Date: ______________________ Fasting Day? Y N

		Macros	
BREAKFAST		Protein	
		Carbs	
		Fat	
		Calories	
LUNCH		Macros	
		Protein	
		Carbs	
		Fat	
		Calories	
DINNER		Macros	
		Protein	
		Carbs	
		Fat	
		Calories	
SNACKS		Macros	
		Protein	
		Carbs	
		Fat	
		Calories	

Hunger / Cravings

None Some Intense

Hydration

Today's Weight

Notes / Observations

Today I Feel...

Sleep Quality

Sleep Time ______

Wake Time ______

z z Z

Date: ______________________ Fasting Day? Y N

		Macros	
BREAKFAST		Protein	
		Carbs	
		Fat	
		Calories	
LUNCH		Macros	
		Protein	
		Carbs	
		Fat	
		Calories	
DINNER		Macros	
		Protein	
		Carbs	
		Fat	
		Calories	
SNACKS		Macros	
		Protein	
		Carbs	
		Fat	
		Calories	

Hunger / Cravings

None Some Intense

Hydration

Today's Weight

Notes / Observations

Today I Feel...

Sleep Quality

Sleep Time ______

Wake Time ______

Date: ____________________ Fasting Day? Y N

		Macros	
BREAKFAST		Protein	
		Carbs	
		Fat	
		Calories	
LUNCH		Macros	
		Protein	
		Carbs	
		Fat	
		Calories	
DINNER		Macros	
		Protein	
		Carbs	
		Fat	
		Calories	
SNACKS		Macros	
		Protein	
		Carbs	
		Fat	
		Calories	

Hunger / Cravings

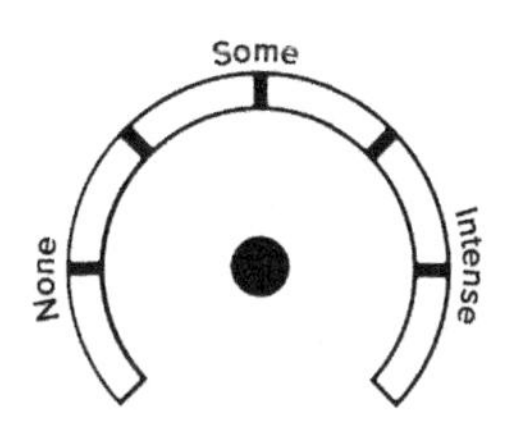

Hydration

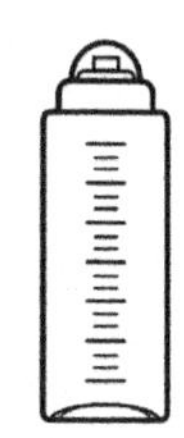

Today's Weight

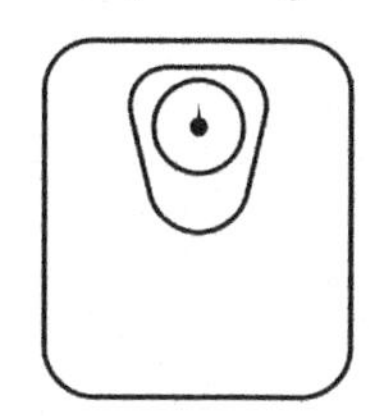

Notes / Observations

Today I Feel...

Sleep Quality

Sleep Time ____________

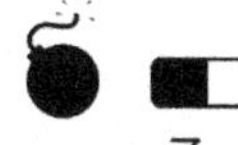
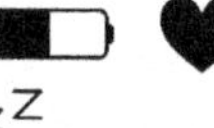

Wake Time ____________

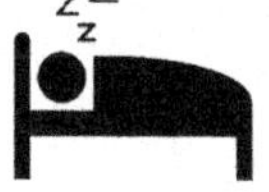

Date: ______________________ Fasting Day? Y N

		Macros	
BREAKFAST		Protein	
		Carbs	
		Fat	
		Calories	
LUNCH		Macros	
		Protein	
		Carbs	
		Fat	
		Calories	
DINNER		Macros	
		Protein	
		Carbs	
		Fat	
		Calories	
SNACKS		Macros	
		Protein	
		Carbs	
		Fat	
		Calories	

Hunger / Cravings

None Some Intense

Hydration

Today's Weight

Notes / Observations

Today I Feel...

Sleep Quality

Sleep Time ______

Wake Time ______

Date: ______________________ Fasting Day? Y N

		Macros	
BREAKFAST		Protein	
		Carbs	
		Fat	
		Calories	
LUNCH		Macros	
		Protein	
		Carbs	
		Fat	
		Calories	
DINNER		Macros	
		Protein	
		Carbs	
		Fat	
		Calories	
SNACKS		Macros	
		Protein	
		Carbs	
		Fat	
		Calories	

Hunger / Cravings

None Some Intense

Hydration

Today's Weight

Notes / Observations

Today I Feel...

Sleep Quality

Sleep Time

Wake Time

Date: ______________________ Fasting Day? Y N

		Macros	
BREAKFAST		Protein	
		Carbs	
		Fat	
		Calories	
LUNCH		Macros	
		Protein	
		Carbs	
		Fat	
		Calories	
DINNER		Macros	
		Protein	
		Carbs	
		Fat	
		Calories	
SNACKS		Macros	
		Protein	
		Carbs	
		Fat	
		Calories	

Hunger / Cravings

None Some Intense

Hydration

Today's Weight

Notes / Observations

Today I Feel...

Sleep Quality

Sleep Time ____________

Wake Time ____________

Date: ______________________ Fasting Day? Y N

		Macros	
BREAKFAST		Protein	
		Carbs	
		Fat	
		Calories	
LUNCH		Macros	
		Protein	
		Carbs	
		Fat	
		Calories	
DINNER		Macros	
		Protein	
		Carbs	
		Fat	
		Calories	
SNACKS		Macros	
		Protein	
		Carbs	
		Fat	
		Calories	

Hunger / Cravings

None Some Intense

Hydration

Today's Weight

Notes / Observations

Today I Feel...

Sleep Quality

Sleep Time ____________

Wake Time ____________

Date: ______________________ Fasting Day? Y N

BREAKFAST		Macros	
		Protein	
		Carbs	
		Fat	
		Calories	
LUNCH		Macros	
		Protein	
		Carbs	
		Fat	
		Calories	
DINNER		Macros	
		Protein	
		Carbs	
		Fat	
		Calories	
SNACKS		Macros	
		Protein	
		Carbs	
		Fat	
		Calories	

Hunger / Cravings

None Some Intense

Hydration

Today's Weight

Notes / Observations

Today I Feel...

Sleep Quality

Sleep Time

Wake Time

Date: ______________________ Fasting Day? Y N

		Macros	
BREAKFAST		Protein	
		Carbs	
		Fat	
		Calories	
		Macros	
LUNCH		Protein	
		Carbs	
		Fat	
		Calories	
		Macros	
DINNER		Protein	
		Carbs	
		Fat	
		Calories	
		Macros	
SNACKS		Protein	
		Carbs	
		Fat	
		Calories	

Hunger / Cravings

None Some Intense

Hydration

Today's Weight

Notes / Observations

Today I Feel...

Sleep Quality

Sleep Time

____

Wake Time

____

Date: ______________________ Fasting Day? Y N

BREAKFAST		MACROS	
		Protein	
		Carbs	
		Fat	
		Calories	
LUNCH		MACROS	
		Protein	
		Carbs	
		Fat	
		Calories	
DINNER		MACROS	
		Protein	
		Carbs	
		Fat	
		Calories	
SNACKS		MACROS	
		Protein	
		Carbs	
		Fat	
		Calories	

Hunger / Cravings

None Some Intense

Hydration

Today's Weight

Notes / Observations

Today I Feel...

Sleep Quality

Sleep Time

Wake Time

Date: ____________________ Fasting Day? Y N

		Macros	
BREAKFAST		Protein	
		Carbs	
		Fat	
		Calories	
		Macros	
LUNCH		Protein	
		Carbs	
		Fat	
		Calories	
		Macros	
DINNER		Protein	
		Carbs	
		Fat	
		Calories	
		Macros	
SNACKS		Protein	
		Carbs	
		Fat	
		Calories	

Hunger / Cravings

None Some Intense

Hydration

Today's Weight

Notes / Observations

....

....

....

....

....

....

....

....

....

....

Today I Feel...

Sleep Quality

Sleep Time ____________

Wake Time ____________

Z z Z

Date: ______________________ Fasting Day? Y N

		MACROS	
BREAKFAST		Protein	
		Carbs	
		Fat	
		Calories	
		MACROS	
LUNCH		Protein	
		Carbs	
		Fat	
		Calories	
		MACROS	
DINNER		Protein	
		Carbs	
		Fat	
		Calories	
		MACROS	
SNACKS		Protein	
		Carbs	
		Fat	
		Calories	

Hunger / Cravings

None Some Intense

Hydration

Today's Weight

Notes / Observations

Today I Feel...

Sleep Quality

Sleep Time ____________

Wake Time ____________

Date: ____________________ Fasting Day? Y N

BREAKFAST		MACROS	
		Protein	
		Carbs	
		Fat	
		Calories	
LUNCH		MACROS	
		Protein	
		Carbs	
		Fat	
		Calories	
DINNER		MACROS	
		Protein	
		Carbs	
		Fat	
		Calories	
SNACKS		MACROS	
		Protein	
		Carbs	
		Fat	
		Calories	

Hunger / Cravings

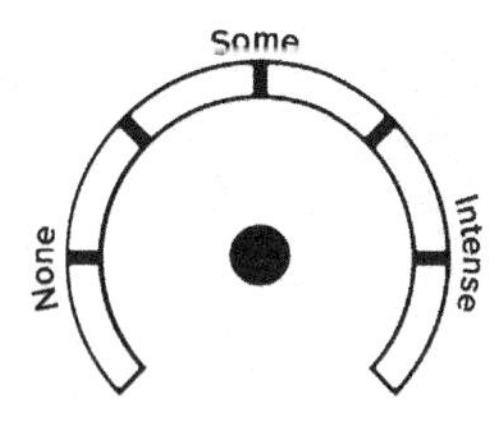

Hydration

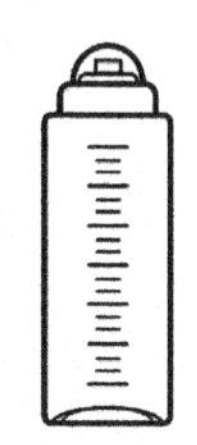

Today's Weight

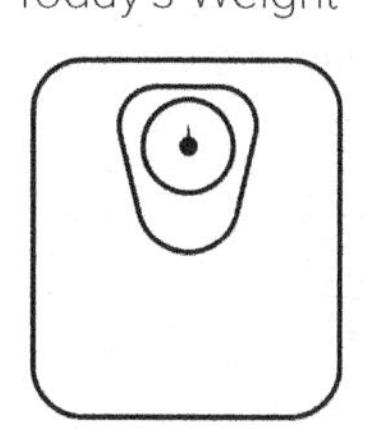

Notes / Observations

....

....

....

....

....

....

....

....

....

....

Today I Feel...

Sleep Quality

Sleep Time ____________

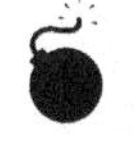
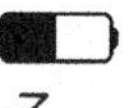

Wake Time ____________

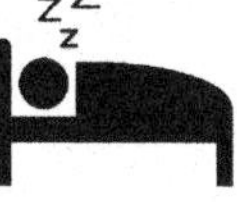

Date: ____________ Fasting Day? Y N

		Macros	
BREAKFAST		Protein	
		Carbs	
		Fat	
		Calories	
LUNCH		Macros	
		Protein	
		Carbs	
		Fat	
		Calories	
DINNER		Macros	
		Protein	
		Carbs	
		Fat	
		Calories	
SNACKS		Macros	
		Protein	
		Carbs	
		Fat	
		Calories	

Hunger / Cravings

None Some Intense

Hydration

Today's Weight

Notes / Observations

Today I Feel...

Sleep Quality

Sleep Time ____________

Wake Time ____________

Date: ______________________ Fasting Day? Y N

BREAKFAST		Macros	
		Protein	
		Carbs	
		Fat	
		Calories	
LUNCH		Macros	
		Protein	
		Carbs	
		Fat	
		Calories	
DINNER		Macros	
		Protein	
		Carbs	
		Fat	
		Calories	
SNACKS		Macros	
		Protein	
		Carbs	
		Fat	
		Calories	

Hunger / Cravings

None Some Intense

Hydration

Today's Weight

Notes / Observations

Today I Feel...

Sleep Quality

Sleep Time

Wake Time

Date: ______________________ Fasting Day? Y N

BREAKFAST		Macros	
		Protein	
		Carbs	
		Fat	
		Calories	
LUNCH		Macros	
		Protein	
		Carbs	
		Fat	
		Calories	
DINNER		Macros	
		Protein	
		Carbs	
		Fat	
		Calories	
SNACKS		Macros	
		Protein	
		Carbs	
		Fat	
		Calories	

Hunger / Cravings

Some

None

Intense

Hydration

Today's Weight

Notes / Observations

Today I Feel...

Sleep Quality

Sleep Time ____________

Wake Time ____________

Date: ______________________ Fasting Day? Y N

		Macros	
BREAKFAST		Protein	
		Carbs	
		Fat	
		Calories	
		Macros	
LUNCH		Protein	
		Carbs	
		Fat	
		Calories	
		Macros	
DINNER		Protein	
		Carbs	
		Fat	
		Calories	
		Macros	
SNACKS		Protein	
		Carbs	
		Fat	
		Calories	

Hunger / Cravings

Some

None

Intense

Hydration

Today's Weight

Notes / Observations

Today I Feel...

Sleep Quality

Sleep Time

____

Wake Time

____

Date: ______________________ Fasting Day? Y N

		Macros	
BREAKFAST		Protein	
		Carbs	
		Fat	
		Calories	
LUNCH		Macros	
		Protein	
		Carbs	
		Fat	
		Calories	
DINNER		Macros	
		Protein	
		Carbs	
		Fat	
		Calories	
SNACKS		Macros	
		Protein	
		Carbs	
		Fat	
		Calories	

Hunger / Cravings

None Some Intense

Hydration

Today's Weight

Notes / Observations

Today I Feel...

Sleep Quality

Sleep Time

Wake Time

Date: ______________________ Fasting Day? Y N

		Macros	
BREAKFAST		Protein	
		Carbs	
		Fat	
		Calories	
LUNCH		Macros	
		Protein	
		Carbs	
		Fat	
		Calories	
DINNER		Macros	
		Protein	
		Carbs	
		Fat	
		Calories	
SNACKS		Macros	
		Protein	
		Carbs	
		Fat	
		Calories	

Hunger / Cravings

None Some Intense

Hydration

Today's Weight

Notes / Observations

Today I Feel...

Sleep Quality

Sleep Time

____

Wake Time

____

Date: ______________________ Fasting Day? Y N

		Macros	
BREAKFAST		Protein	
		Carbs	
		Fat	
		Calories	
LUNCH		Macros	
		Protein	
		Carbs	
		Fat	
		Calories	
DINNER		Macros	
		Protein	
		Carbs	
		Fat	
		Calories	
SNACKS		Macros	
		Protein	
		Carbs	
		Fat	
		Calories	

Hunger / Cravings

None Some Intense

Hydration

Today's Weight

Notes / Observations

Today I Feel...

Sleep Quality

Sleep Time

Wake Time

Date: ____________________ Fasting Day? Y N

BREAKFAST		Macros	
		Protein	
		Carbs	
		Fat	
		Calories	
LUNCH		Macros	
		Protein	
		Carbs	
		Fat	
		Calories	
DINNER		Macros	
		Protein	
		Carbs	
		Fat	
		Calories	
SNACKS		Macros	
		Protein	
		Carbs	
		Fat	
		Calories	

Hunger / Cravings

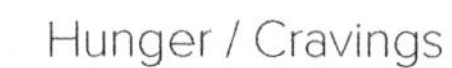

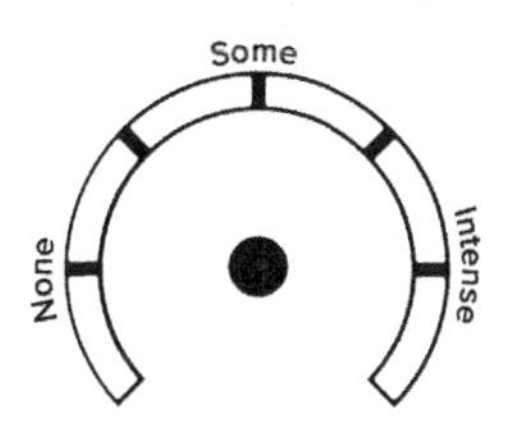

Hydration

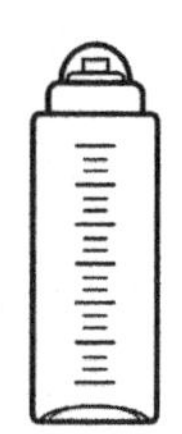

Today's Weight

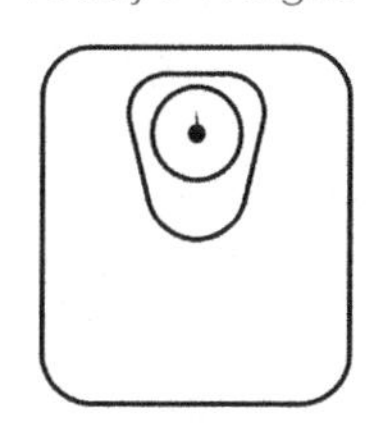

Notes / Observations

....

....

....

....

....

....

....

....

....

....

Today I Feel...

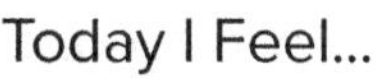

Sleep Quality

Sleep Time

____

Wake Time

____

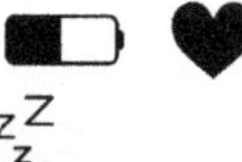

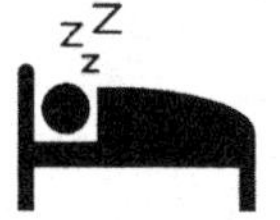

Date: ______________ Fasting Day? Y N

		Macros	
BREAKFAST		Protein	
		Carbs	
		Fat	
		Calories	
LUNCH		Macros	
		Protein	
		Carbs	
		Fat	
		Calories	
DINNER		Macros	
		Protein	
		Carbs	
		Fat	
		Calories	
SNACKS		Macros	
		Protein	
		Carbs	
		Fat	
		Calories	

Hunger / Cravings

None Some Intense

Hydration

Today's Weight

Notes / Observations

Today I Feel...

Sleep Quality

Sleep Time ______________

Wake Time ______________

Date: ______________________ Fasting Day? Y N

		Macros	
BREAKFAST		Protein	
		Carbs	
		Fat	
		Calories	
LUNCH		Macros	
		Protein	
		Carbs	
		Fat	
		Calories	
DINNER		Macros	
		Protein	
		Carbs	
		Fat	
		Calories	
SNACKS		Macros	
		Protein	
		Carbs	
		Fat	
		Calories	

Hunger / Cravings

None Some Intense

Hydration

Today's Weight

Notes / Observations

Today I Feel...

Sleep Quality

Sleep Time ______

Wake Time ______

Date: ______________________ Fasting Day? Y N

		Macros	
Breakfast		Protein	
		Carbs	
		Fat	
		Calories	
		Macros	
Lunch		Protein	
		Carbs	
		Fat	
		Calories	
		Macros	
Dinner		Protein	
		Carbs	
		Fat	
		Calories	
		Macros	
Snacks		Protein	
		Carbs	
		Fat	
		Calories	

Hunger / Cravings

None Some Intense

Hydration

Today's Weight

Notes / Observations

Today I Feel...

Sleep Quality

Sleep Time

____

Wake Time

____

Date: ______________________ Fasting Day? Y N

		Macros	
BREAKFAST		Protein	
		Carbs	
		Fat	
		Calories	
LUNCH		Macros	
		Protein	
		Carbs	
		Fat	
		Calories	
DINNER		Macros	
		Protein	
		Carbs	
		Fat	
		Calories	
SNACKS		Macros	
		Protein	
		Carbs	
		Fat	
		Calories	

Hunger / Cravings

None Some Intense

Hydration

Today's Weight

Notes / Observations

Today I Feel...

Sleep Quality

Sleep Time

____

Wake Time

____

Date: ______________________ Fasting Day? Y N

		Macros	
BREAKFAST		Protein	
		Carbs	
		Fat	
		Calories	
LUNCH		Macros	
		Protein	
		Carbs	
		Fat	
		Calories	
DINNER		Macros	
		Protein	
		Carbs	
		Fat	
		Calories	
SNACKS		Macros	
		Protein	
		Carbs	
		Fat	
		Calories	

Hunger / Cravings

None Some Intense

Hydration

Today's Weight

Notes / Observations

Today I Feel...

Sleep Quality

Sleep Time ____________

Wake Time ____________

Date: ____________________ Fasting Day? Y N

		Macros	
BREAKFAST		Protein	
		Carbs	
		Fat	
		Calories	
LUNCH		Macros	
		Protein	
		Carbs	
		Fat	
		Calories	
DINNER		Macros	
		Protein	
		Carbs	
		Fat	
		Calories	
SNACKS		Macros	
		Protein	
		Carbs	
		Fat	
		Calories	

Hunger / Cravings

None Some Intense

Hydration

Today's Weight

Notes / Observations

Today I Feel...

Sleep Quality

Sleep Time

Wake Time

Date: ______________________ Fasting Day? Y N

BREAKFAST		Macros	
		Protein	
		Carbs	
		Fat	
		Calories	
LUNCH		Macros	
		Protein	
		Carbs	
		Fat	
		Calories	
DINNER		Macros	
		Protein	
		Carbs	
		Fat	
		Calories	
SNACKS		Macros	
		Protein	
		Carbs	
		Fat	
		Calories	

Hunger / Cravings

None Some Intense

Hydration

Today's Weight

Notes / Observations

Today I Feel...

Sleep Quality

Sleep Time

Wake Time

Date: ______________________ Fasting Day? Y N

		Macros	
BREAKFAST		Protein	
		Carbs	
		Fat	
		Calories	
LUNCH		Macros	
		Protein	
		Carbs	
		Fat	
		Calories	
DINNER		Macros	
		Protein	
		Carbs	
		Fat	
		Calories	
SNACKS		Macros	
		Protein	
		Carbs	
		Fat	
		Calories	

Hunger / Cravings

None Some Intense

Hydration

Today's Weight

Notes / Observations

Today I Feel...

Sleep Quality

Sleep Time

Wake Time

Date: ____________________ Fasting Day? Y N

BREAKFAST		Macros	
		Protein	
		Carbs	
		Fat	
		Calories	
LUNCH		Macros	
		Protein	
		Carbs	
		Fat	
		Calories	
DINNER		Macros	
		Protein	
		Carbs	
		Fat	
		Calories	
SNACKS		Macros	
		Protein	
		Carbs	
		Fat	
		Calories	

Hunger / Cravings

None Some Intense

Hydration

Today's Weight

Notes / Observations

Today I Feel...

Sleep Quality

Sleep Time ____________

Wake Time ____________

Date: ______________________ Fasting Day? Y N

		Macros	
BREAKFAST		Protein	
		Carbs	
		Fat	
		Calories	
LUNCH		Macros	
		Protein	
		Carbs	
		Fat	
		Calories	
DINNER		Macros	
		Protein	
		Carbs	
		Fat	
		Calories	
SNACKS		Macros	
		Protein	
		Carbs	
		Fat	
		Calories	

Hunger / Cravings

None Some Intense

Hydration

Today's Weight

Notes / Observations

Today I Feel...

Sleep Quality

Sleep Time ______

Wake Time ______

Made in the USA
Middletown, DE
08 August 2023